ANDRE'S ARMOR

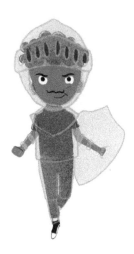

Story by: Dr. Mohamed "Mo" Jalloh   Illustrated: by Gabriel Lopez

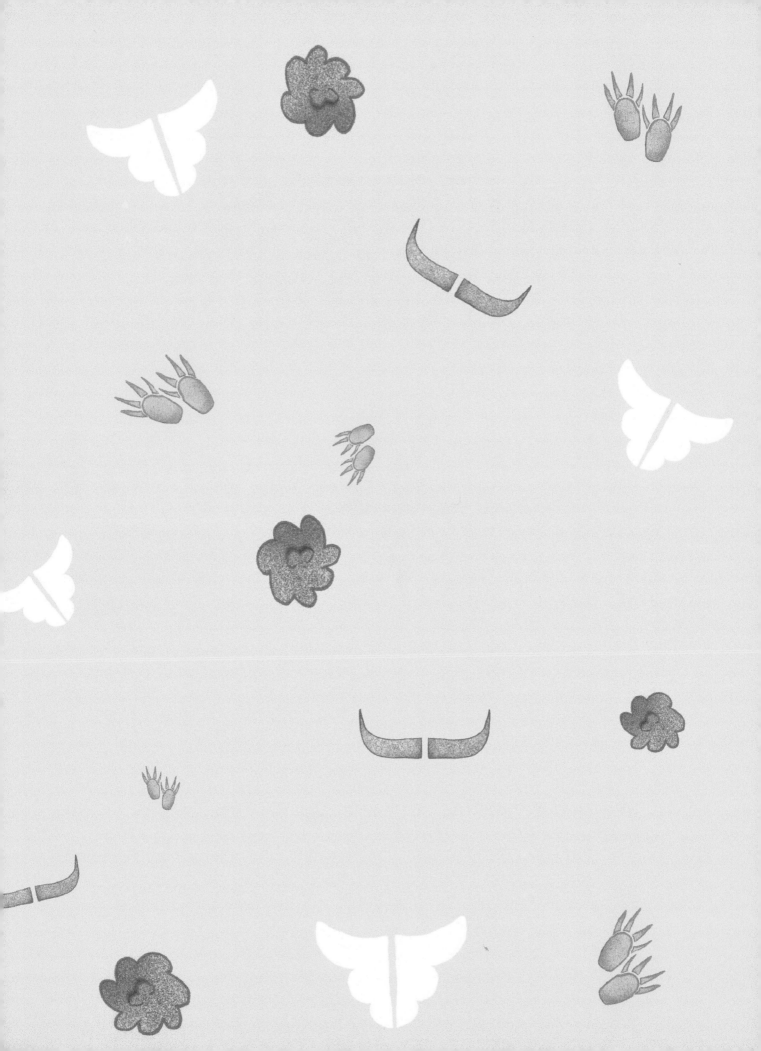

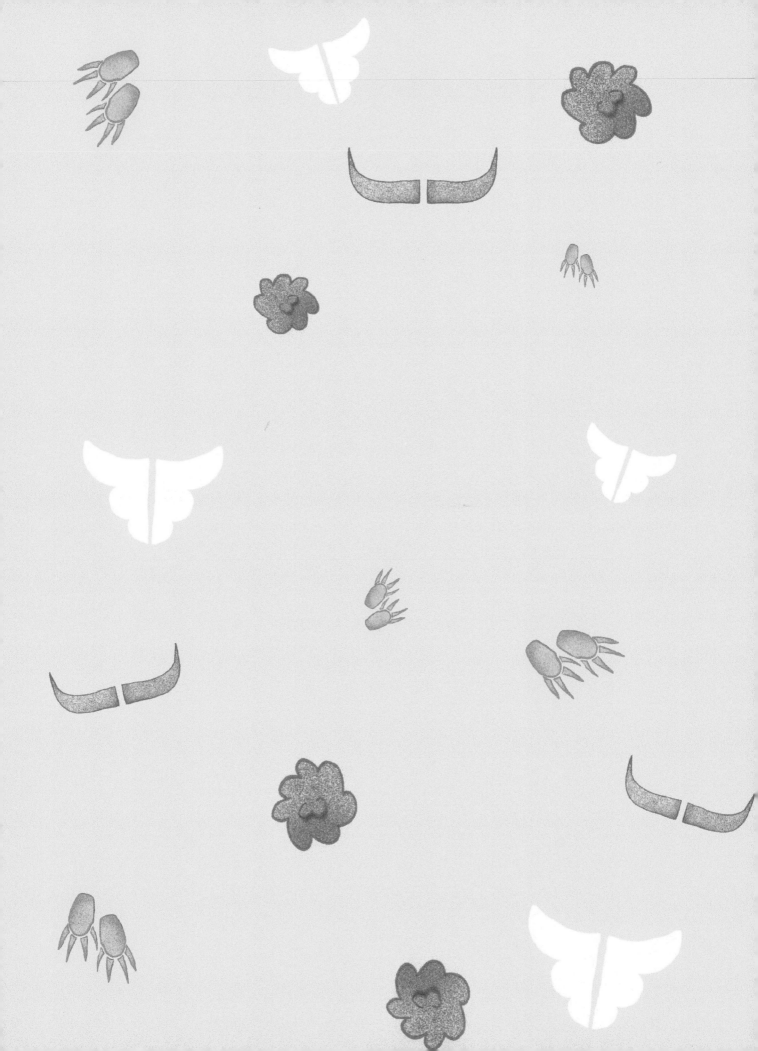

ISBN: 978-0-578-94565-1

For Mom, Sue, and Kadija. May your love and support continue to provide comfort to all of us young kids when we get all of the different shots in our lives—M.J.

Andre and his mom were waiting to be seen at the doctor's for his shots.

Andre was playing a video game fighting against some monster bots.

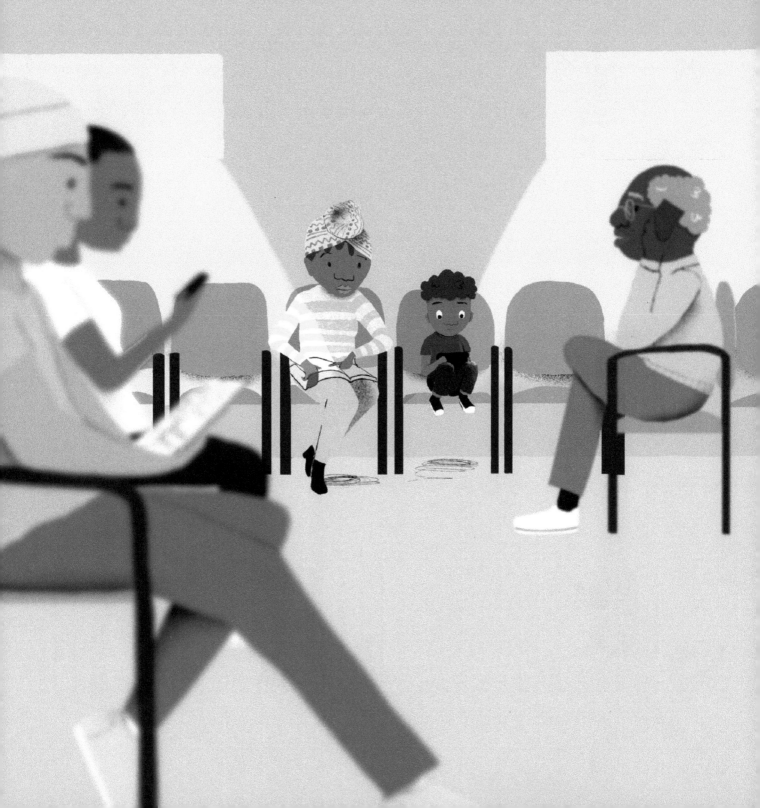

He was just about to level up to Castle Zone 22,

When suddenly he heard, "Andre, the doctor's ready for you."

Andre looked up fearfully - he didn't want a shot.

The *doctor* might be ready, Andre thought, but *I* am not!

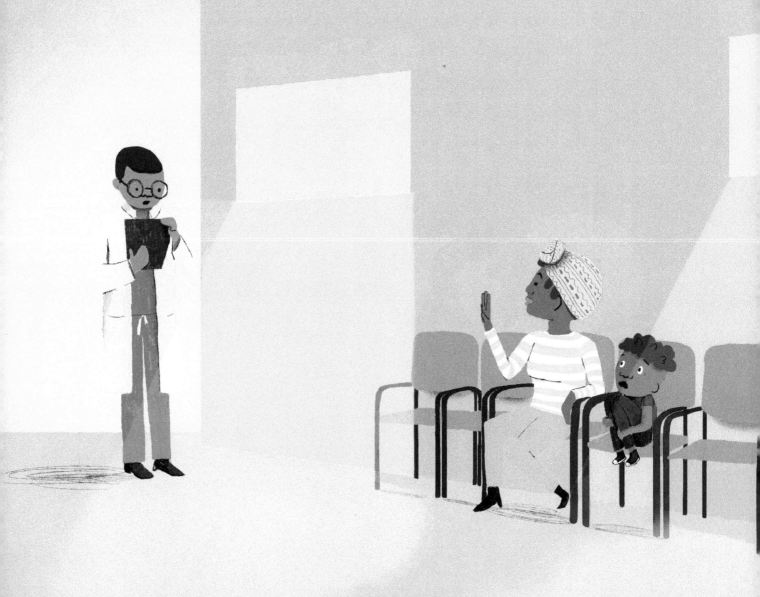

Andre tried to run……

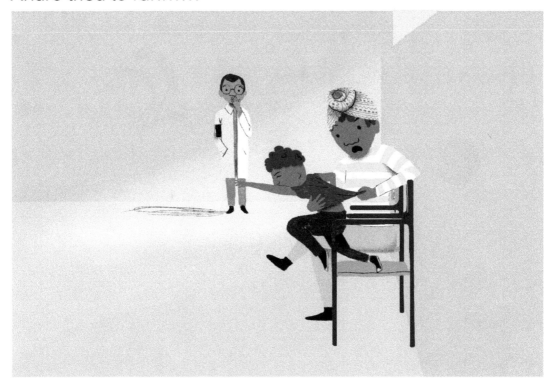

Andre tried to hide…..

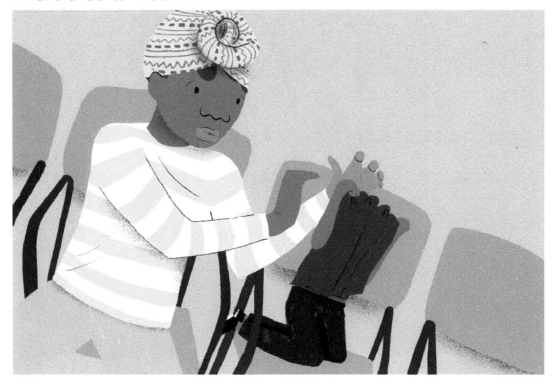

But, his mother reassured him, "Shots protect us from inside."

"I really want you to be safe. No need to hide."

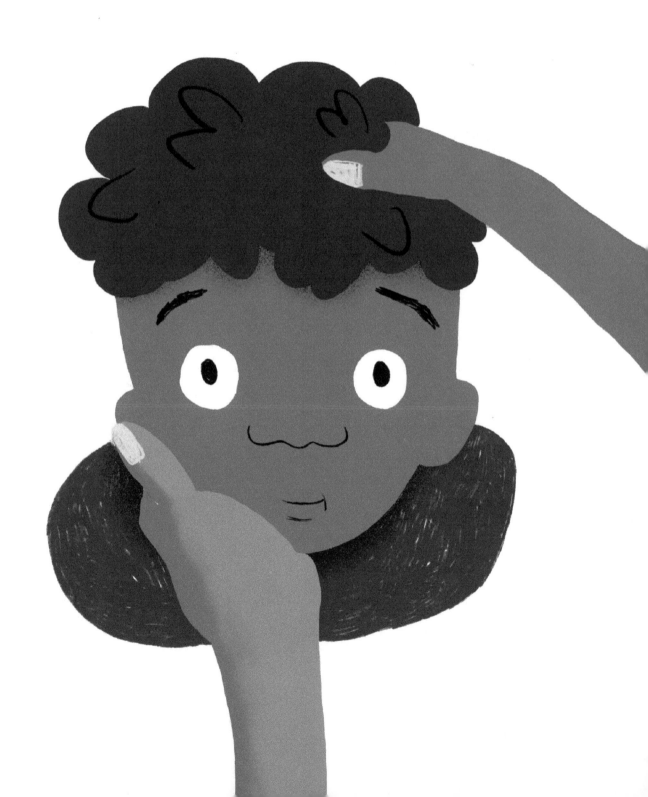

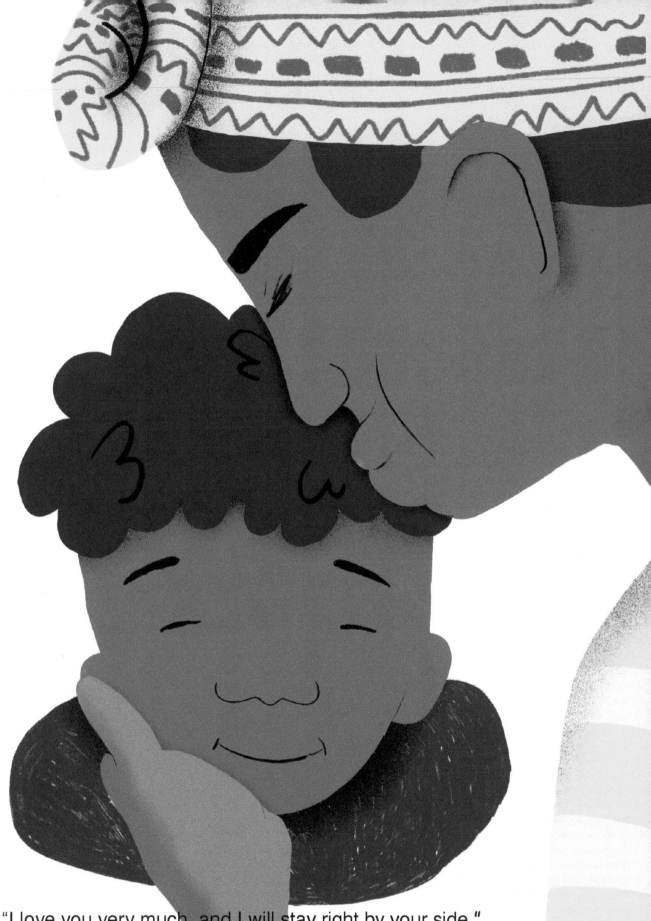

"I love you very much, and I will stay right by your side."

Dr. Okafor walked in to see her favorite little patient.

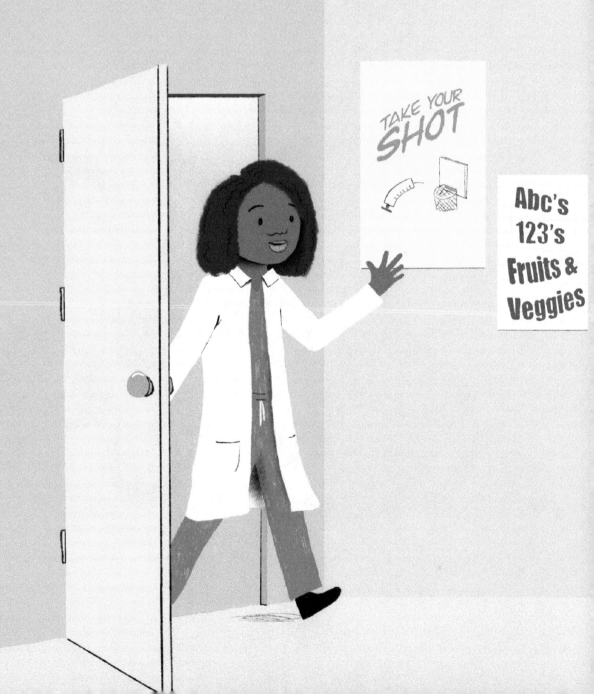

Andre was busy playing with her stethescope - it looked so old and ancient.

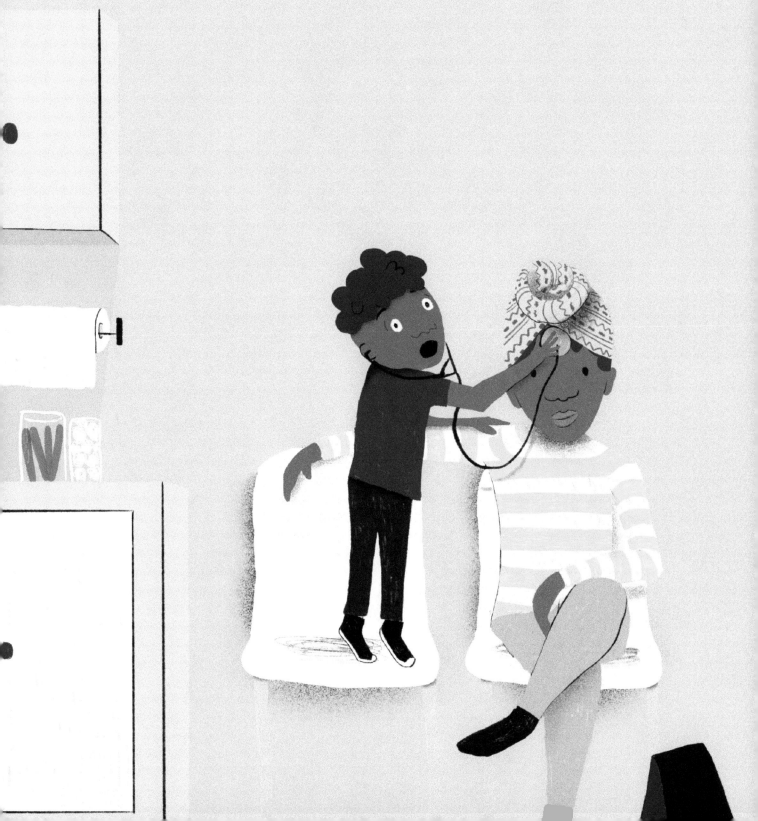

Again, Andre tried to run…

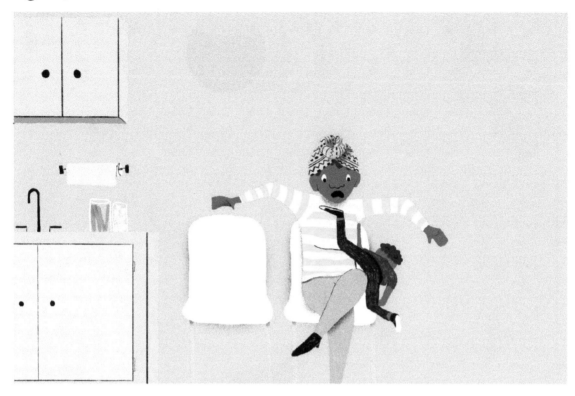

Andre tried to hide…..

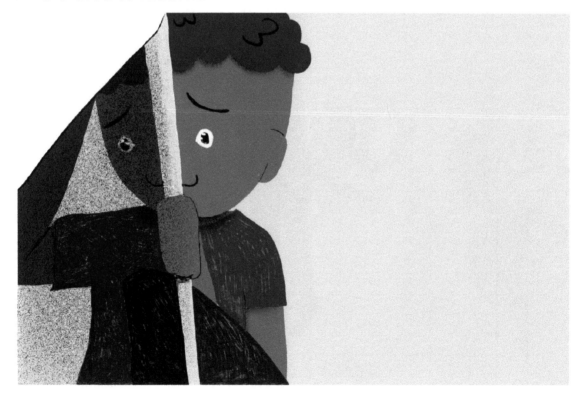

Dr. Okafor could tell that Andre was scared inside.

"Aww, lil buddy, what's the matter? Why are you afraid?"

But Andre only whimpered, 'til his mom came to his aid.

"He's scared to get his shots," she said. "He doesn't think they're cool.

But we know he needs them before he starts going to school."

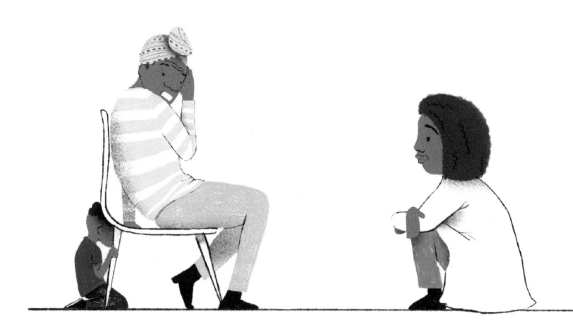

Andre asked, "Why do I have to get that scary thing?"

"I heard that they hurt and don't do anything!"

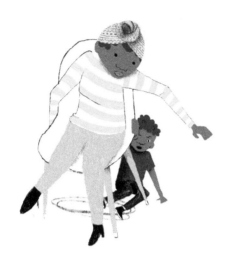

"If you ask me, shots sound very boring, dumb, and lame."

"I just wanna play my Monster vs Knights video game!"

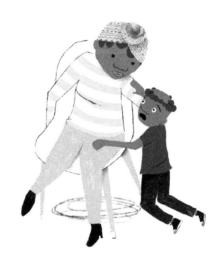

Dr. Okafor thought hard. She saw Andre was upset.

How could she explain that shots are fun and cool to get?

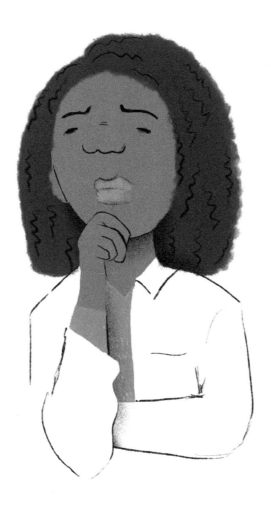

"I got it!" Dr. Okafor said. "How about I explain to you...

...exactly what these shots are made to do?

They make sure you don't get sick - like knights getting power ups and shields."

This made Andre think back to his video game with all of the monsters in the fields.

Dr. Okafor then drew several pictures using color and detail

Andre listened curiously to her exciting, new tale.

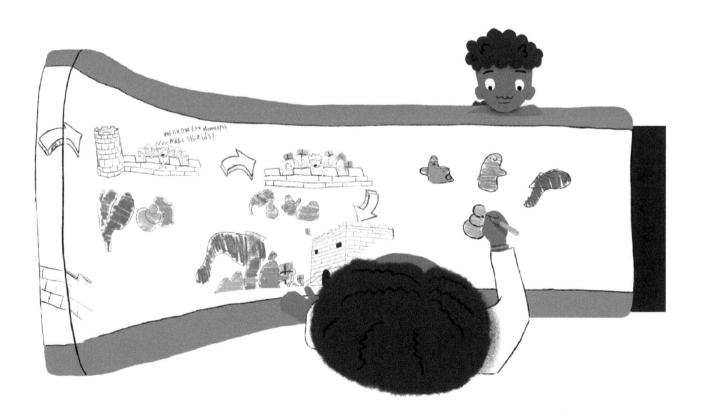

"Each shot is like an eagle carrying an important message to a king of your body or your castle.

The message teaches your body what germ monsters to watch for without too much hassle."

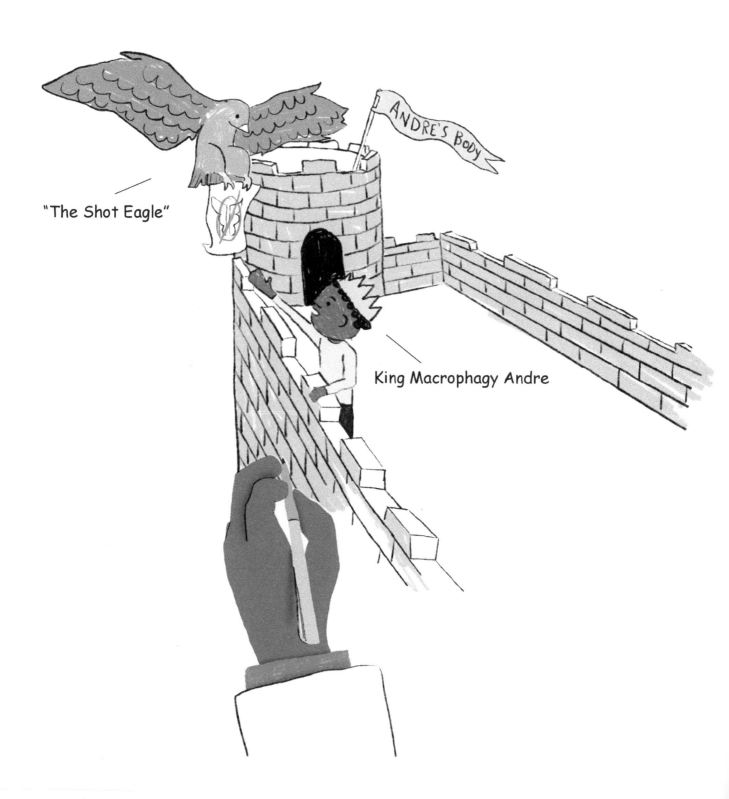

"The Shot Eagle"

King Macrophagy Andre

This message says that "germs with wings are not welcome in your kingdom.

Your king must now warn his knights about this newly delivered wisdom."

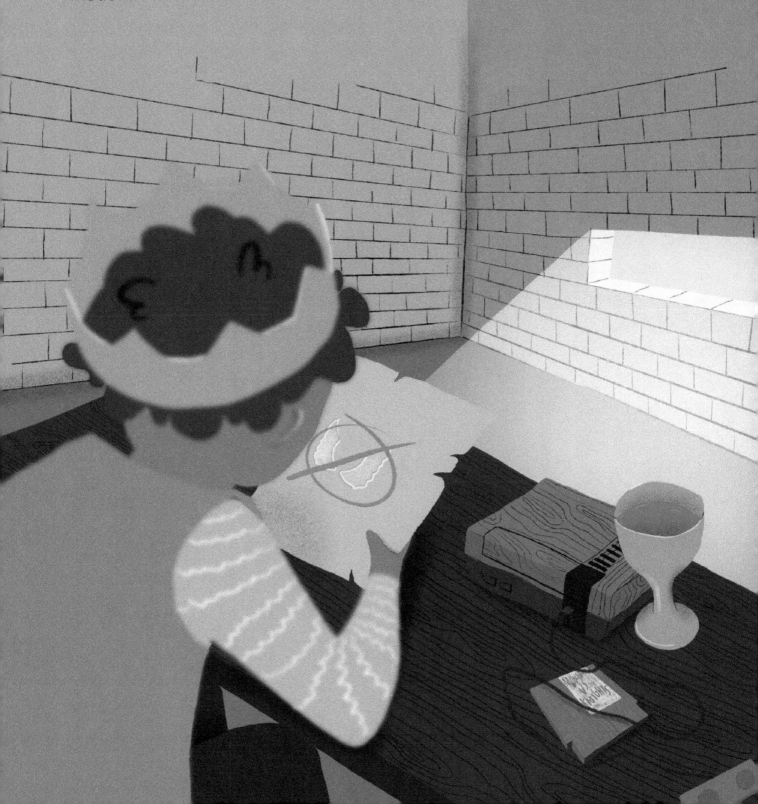

Your kingdom's best protectors are the White Blood Cell Knights.

The king commands them, "Fight any germ with these wings with all of your might!"

Andre's White Blood Cell Armor Knights

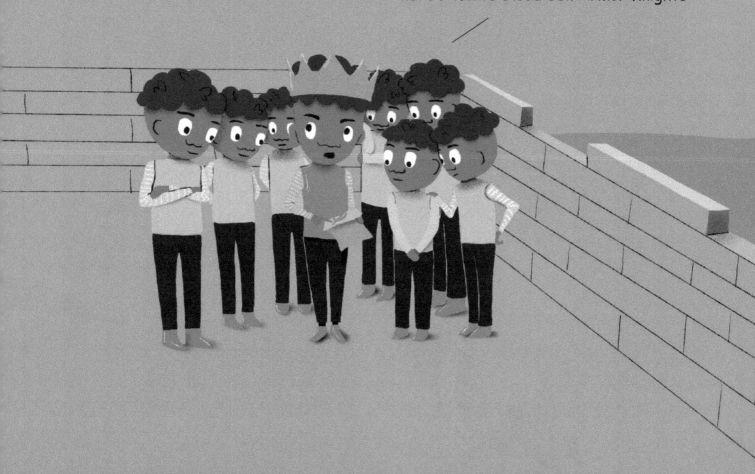

"Soon the knights build antibody armor and shields, among other things...

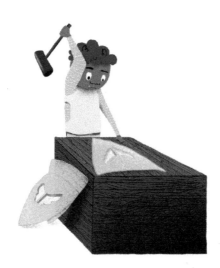

To keep their kingdom - that's your body - safe from germs with wings!"

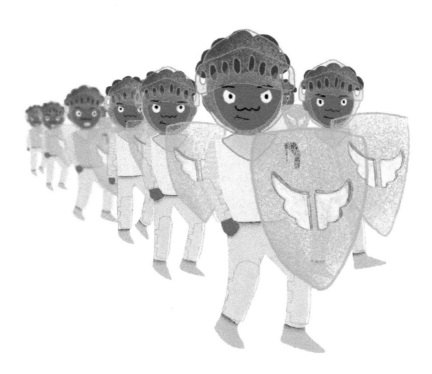

That way, if ever the winged-germ monsters try to attack young Andre's castle.

They're sure to get a big surprise - all of the knights wearing armor built to dazzle.

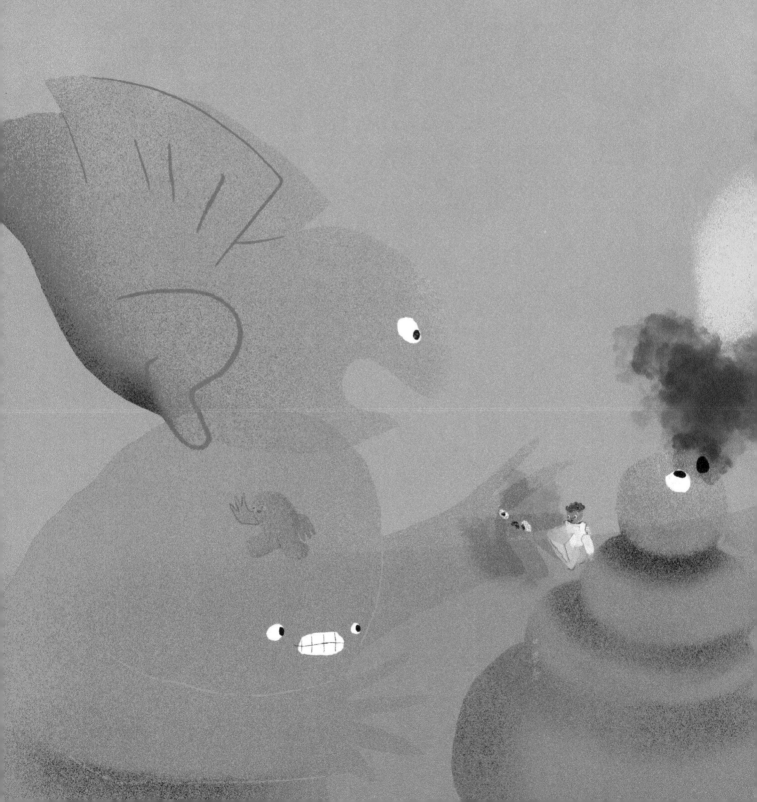

The knights are easily armed to defend Andre from scary germs that come his way.

The new armor will cause all of the winged-germ monsters to take one look and fly away.

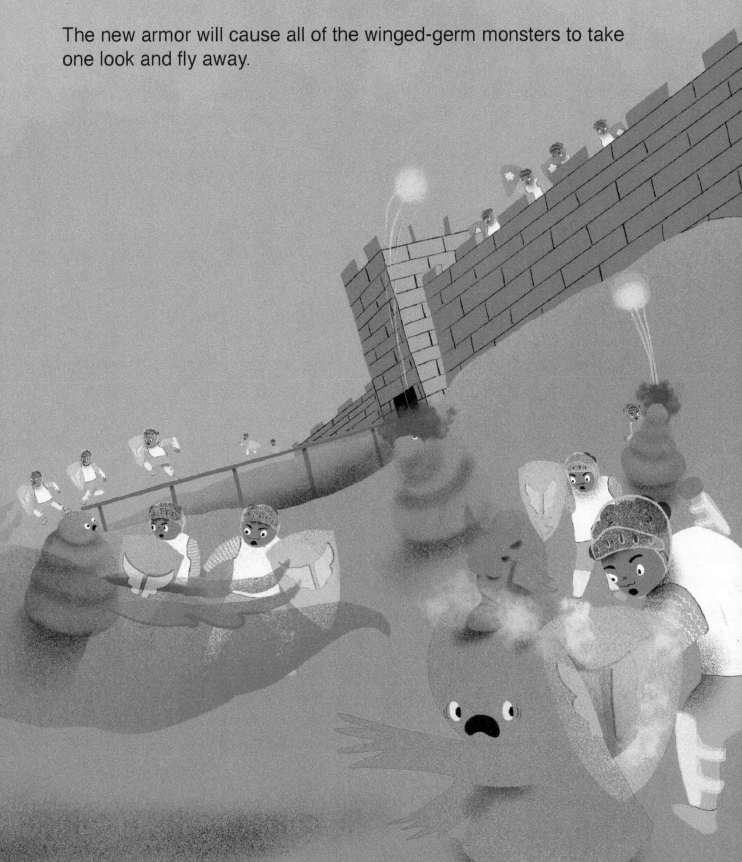

Andre thought that his body's king and knights were very cool.

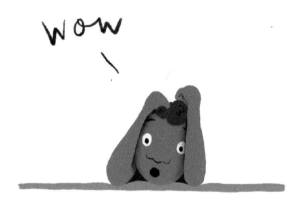

"But wait," he said. "Why do I have to get so many shots for school?"

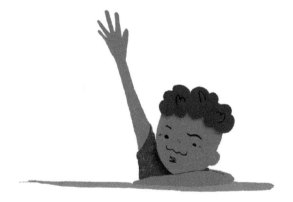

Dr. Okafor explained, "*Some* germs have claws, horns, *or even* spit fireballs.

We've got to prep your body to protect your castle walls!"

"Now, let me test you, so let's say we want to teach your body how to protect itself from green germs with wings...

....and teach it to be protected from some blue germs who spit fireballs that even sting.

Tell me, Andre, what do you think we ought to do?

The red shot, blue shot or the green shot? Which armors should I give to you?"

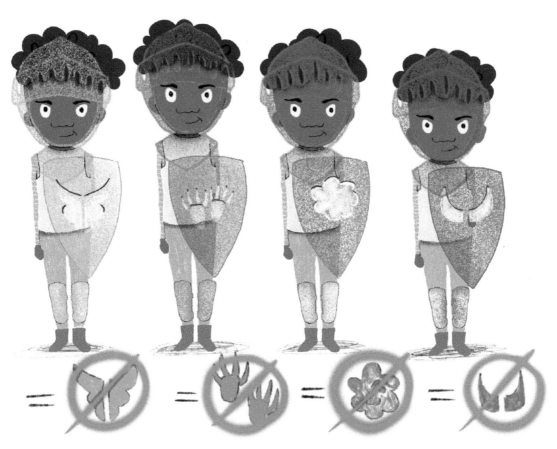

He looked back at the castle pictures and he had no doubt.

"I wanna get the green one *and* the blue one," Andre shouts.

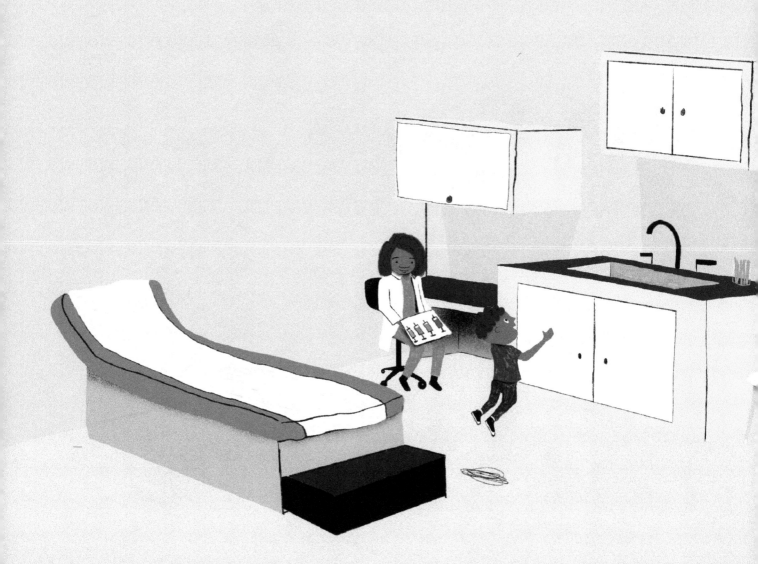

Dr. Okafor said, "Good job Andre! Those are the best to get!

Now your body will fight both of those germs and won't forget!"

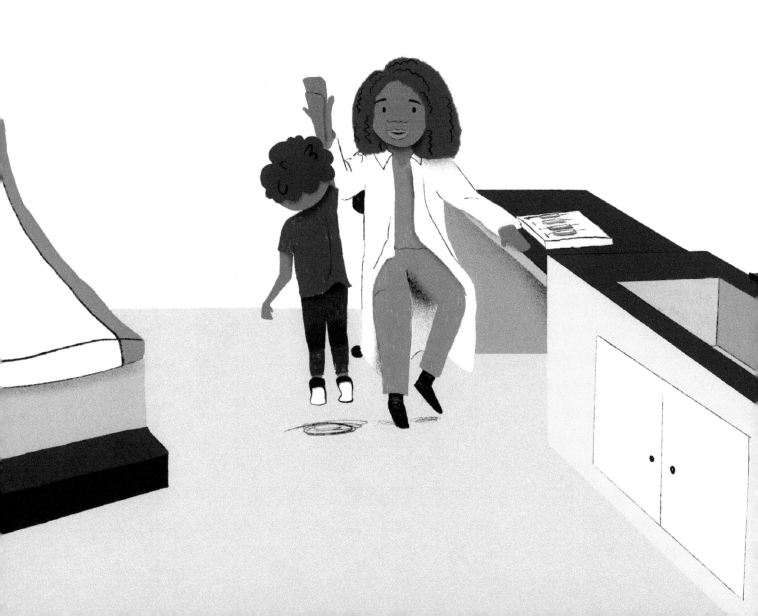

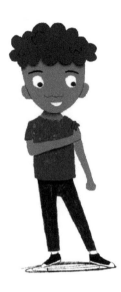

"Uhm, how do we know they will work and do what they are gonna do?"

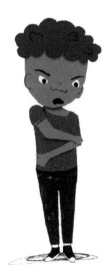

Andre's mom said, "Good question, Dre! Please Doc, I want to know that too!"

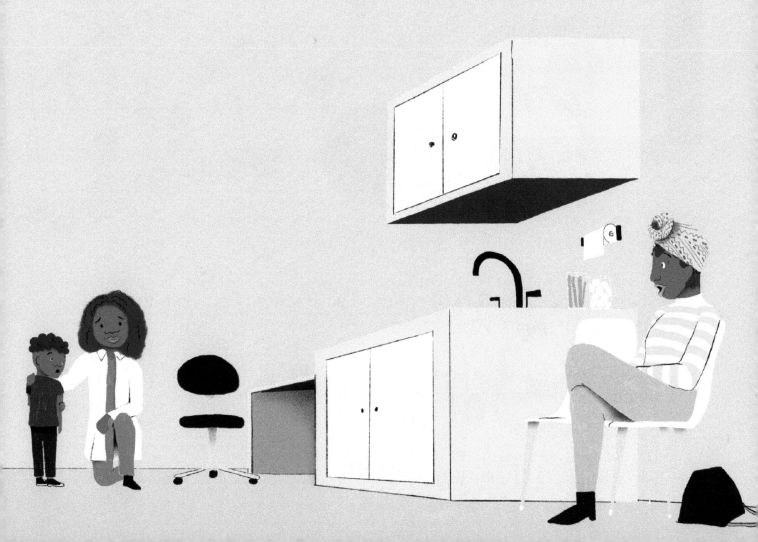

"Well a shot is tested in the lab for a long time," Dr. Okafor said.

"Then it is tested with some kids to make sure they don't get sick and have to stay home in bed.

Then some smart people get together and see whether they should let other kids get this shot too.

I can only give you this shot if the smart people agree that they work to protect kids from yucky germ monsters. *Ewww*!!!"

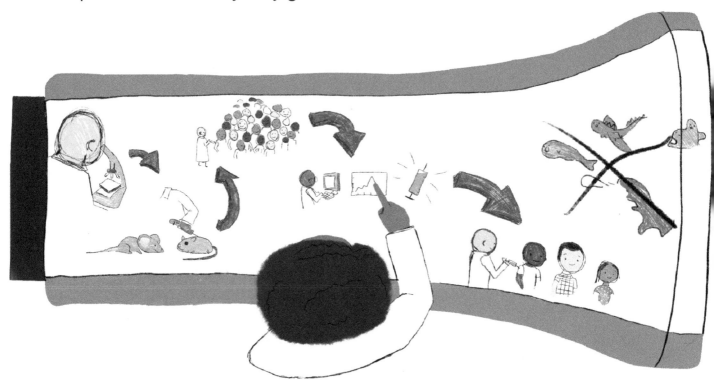

"Guess what, mom? I just checked your records and see that you are due for one of *your* shots too.

Would you like to get your shot with Andre, to make sure your castle is also protected through and through?"

"Yay Mom!" Andre smiled. "Let's both protect our castles."

"Of course, Dre! Let's protect both of our bodies with no hassle."

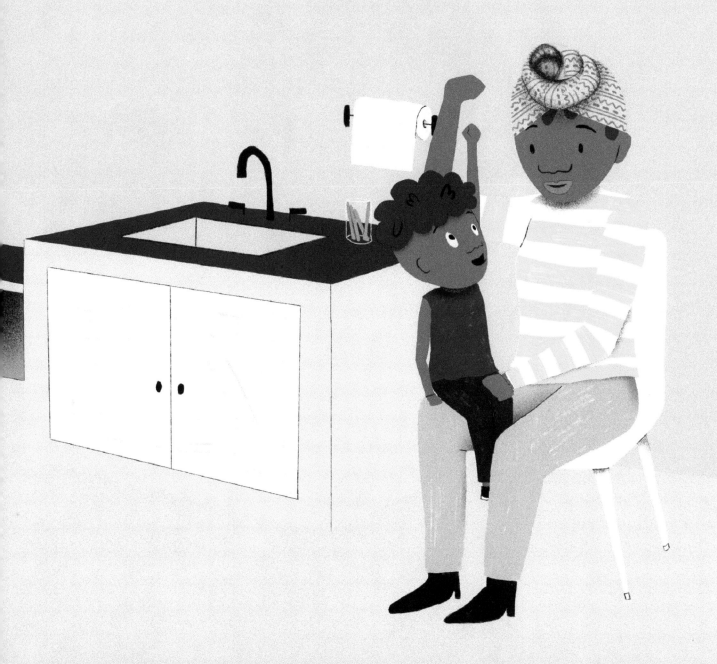

Dr. Okafor gave Andre his shots, green and blue.

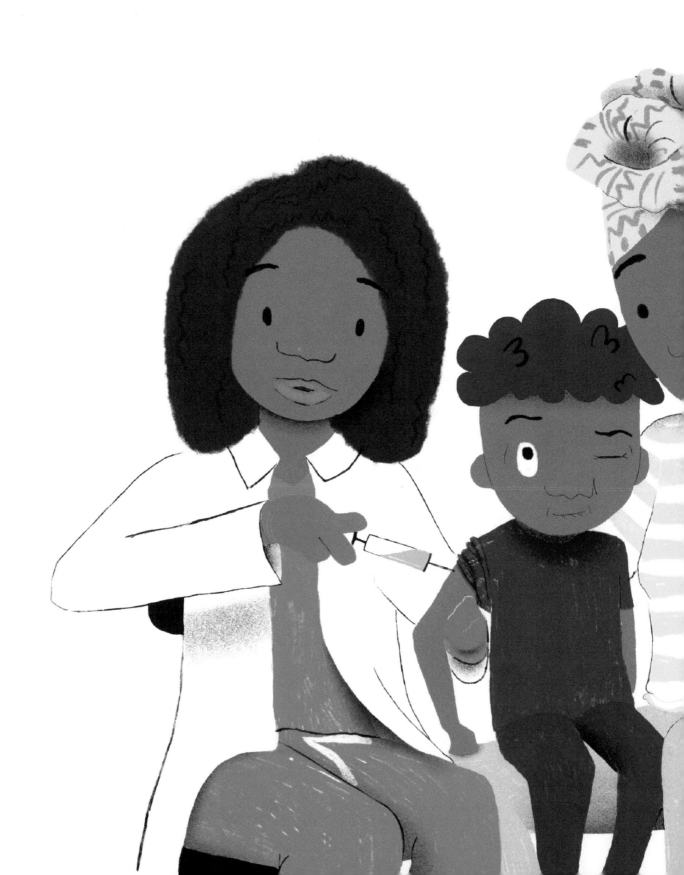

Then she gave his mother her shot - the red one too!

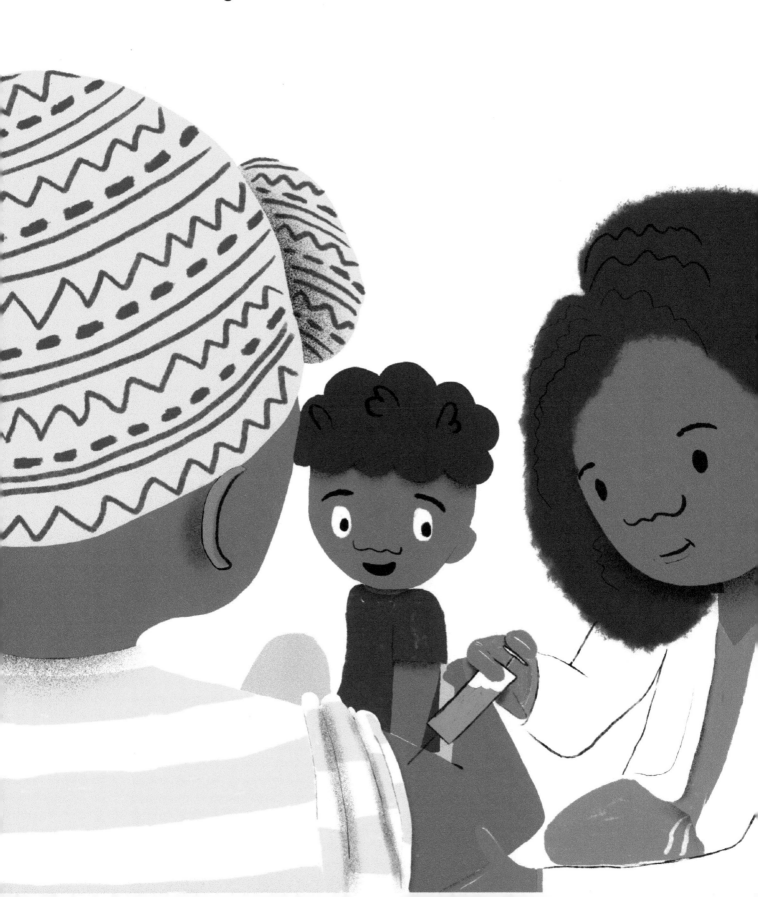

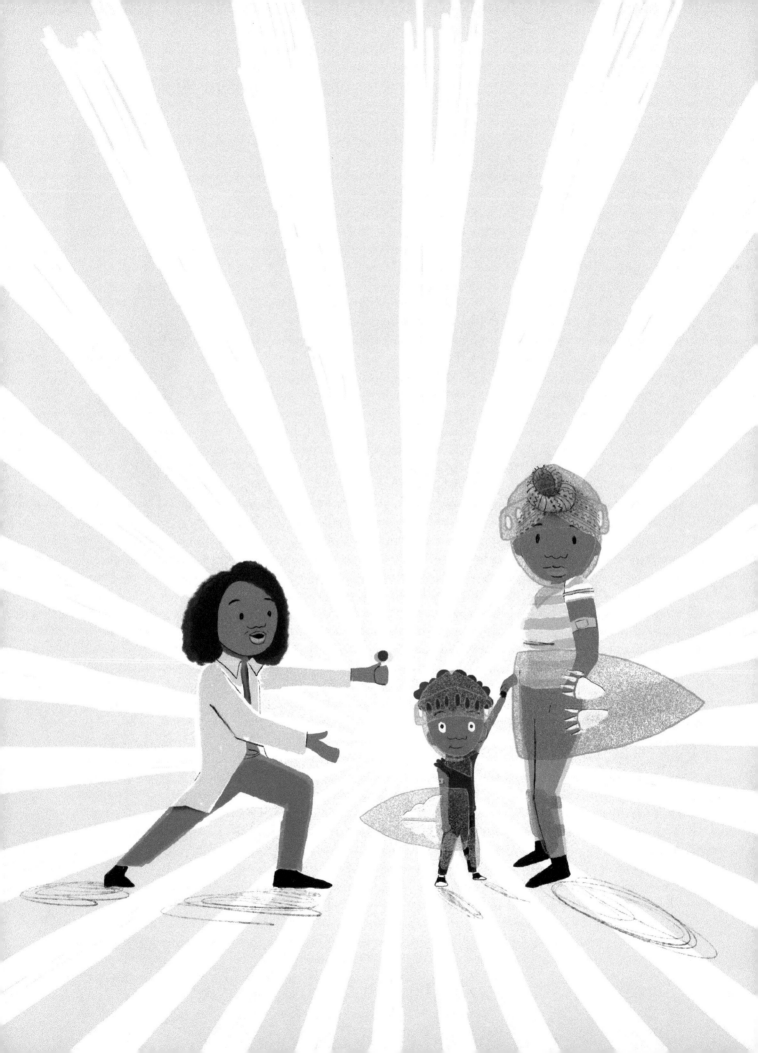

"Bye-Bye, Andre. And good luck this coming year in school.

You will be protected from those germ monsters, how cool!"

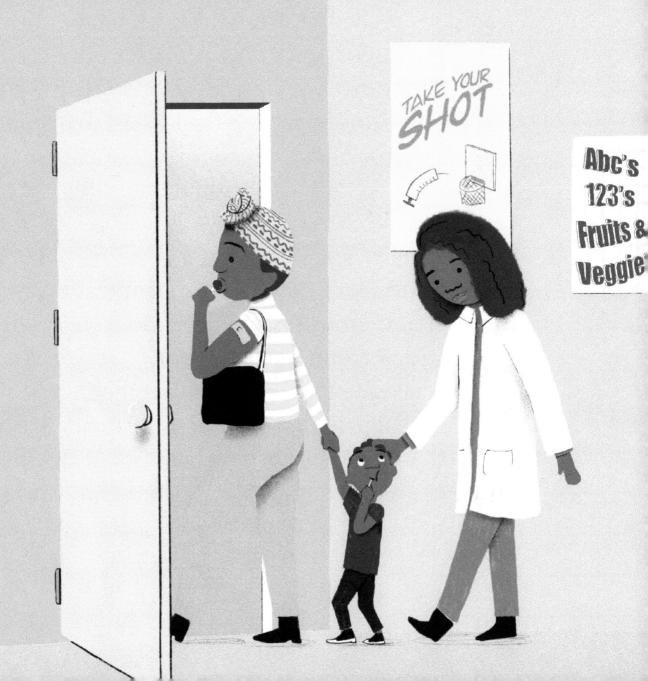

"Thank you for reading this book to a child! The goal of this book is to empower parents and caregivers to be more informed about how vaccines work so they can make better informed decisions. Vaccines are one of the greatest medical success stories in history. Before vaccines, many people would get really sick from diseases such as polio and smallpox since yucky viruses or bacteria would easily invade our body. Vaccines are synthetic photocopies of specific parts of a virus and they teach our body to recognize that part to protect against. When the virus returns, after we have received a vaccine, our body knows how to identify, neutralize and eliminate it right away. Luckily before vaccines are available to people, they go through numerous tests to verify that they work. Afterward, a group of world renowned experts review that data to make sure that they work. Once a vaccine is approved or authorized by such experts, then parents can feel confident that their children are receiving a safe vaccine that works."

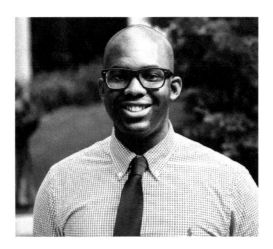

Dr. Mohamed Jalloh (@DrMohamedRx) is a children's book author with a passion for teaching young kids how medicines work. He has a Doctor of Pharmacy degree (Pharm.D.) and has spent many years in the medical field treating patients in a family medicine clinic, giving vaccines at pharmacies, and teaching students. He hopes to inspire minority children to pursue an education in healthcare.

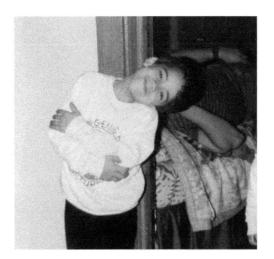

Gabriel Lopez is a curious creative living in Chicago with his wife and son. You can find Gabriel in his home office producing music and drawing pictures, with this being his fourth picture book.
Gabriel doesn't like getting shots, but loves how cool he'd look in that red armor.

www.gabriellopez.co

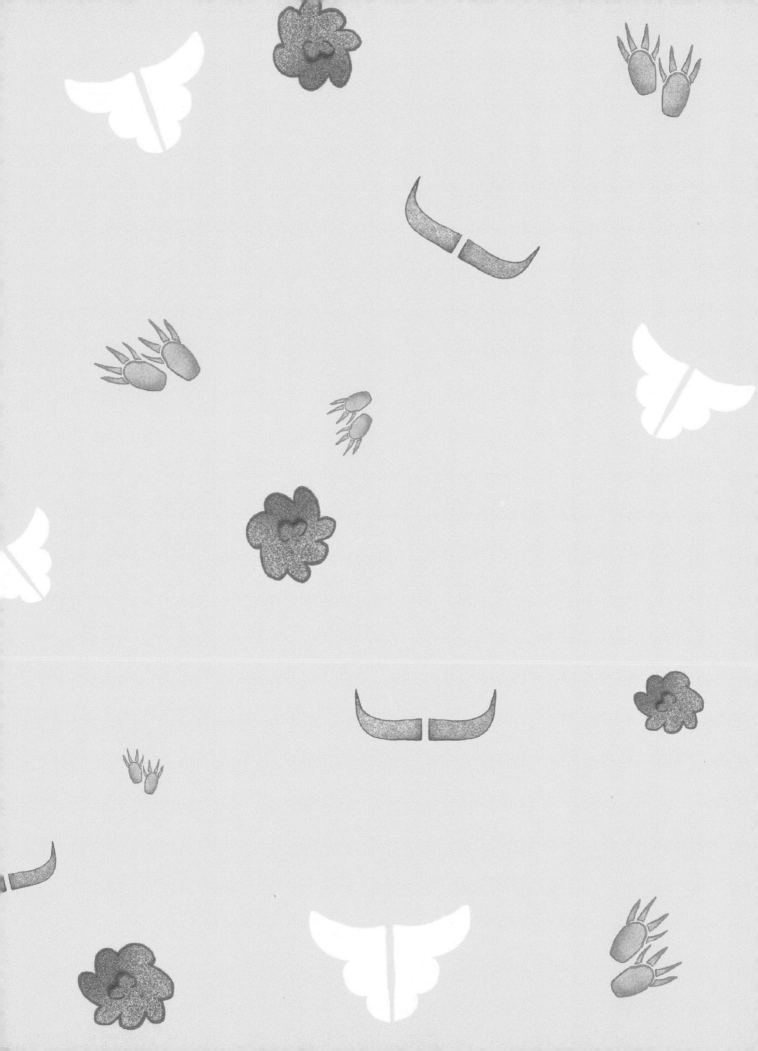